# Homœopathy
## for
# Emergencies

# Homoeopathy for Emergencies

## PHYLLIS SPEIGHT

Health Science Press
The C.W. Daniel Company Ltd
1 Church Path, Saffron Walden, Essex, England

First published in Great Britain by
The C.W. Daniel Company Limited
1 Church Path, Saffron Walden,
Essex, England

© Phyllis Speight 1984

Reprinted 1990

ISBN 0 85207 162 0

Set in 10pt Melior 2pt leaded by
Simpson Typesetting, Bishop's Stortford

The Random House Group Limited supports The Forest Stewardship
Council (FSC®), the leading international forest certification organisation.
Our books carrying the FSC label are printed on FSC® certified paper.
FSC is the only forest certification scheme endorsed by the leading
environmental organisations, including Greenpeace. Our
paper procurement policy can be found at
www.randomhouse.co.uk/environment

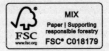

MIX
Paper | Supporting
responsible forestry
FSC® C018179

Printed and bound in Great Britain by Clays Ltd, St Ives PLC

# CONTENTS

# INTRODUCTION

This small book has been written to enable those with no knowledge of homoeopathy to apply the remedies in emergencies and injuries.

These are safe and have no side effects and if well chosen to match the patient's symptoms they can produce amazing results.

The emergencies are listed in alphabetical order and I have tried to include anything that can develop quickly and needs prompt attention. In some cases a doctor should be called but, even so, help may be given pending his arrival.

Obviously it has been necessary to limit the number of remedies and in certain cases the appropriate medicines may not be included. However, those named will assist in the majority of cases.

I suggest that anyone who is really interested in homoeopathy should study some of the books recommended on page 57.

The remedies given for injuries and first-aid are specifics but when dealing with acute conditions the medicine should be selected to match the symptoms of the patient.

To do this it is helpful to write down the answers as follows:

Location = The exact position of the trouble.
Sensation = The feeling experienced, e.g. heat, cold, throbbing, soreness etc.
Modalities = Anything that makes the symptom(s) better or

worse, e.g. heat, cold, position, pressure, movement etc.

Cause, if known = This can be useful.

In section 2 the main characteristics of remedies are given because they are helpful and enable the prescriber to differentiate. Many remedies have symptoms in common but the selection can often be simplified by a reference to their individual characteristics.

**Phyllis Speight**

# Please read this – it is important!

## POTENCIES AND DOSAGE

The following is an explanation of both potency and dose as both can be very confusing.

Homoeopathic remedies are available in an almost unlimited range of potencies which all work when correctly prescribed. There are, however, some factors which must be taken into account when deciding upon the most suitable potency which controls the dosage.

An understanding of the way in which potencies are prepared should help to clarify the problem.

Potentisation is a simple process whereby one drop of the original substance (mother tincture) [indicated by $\emptyset$ in the text] is added to ninety nine drops of diluent (usually distilled water) and vigorously shaken about thirty times. This gives the first centesimal potency which is indicated by the number 1 (sometimes 1c) following the name of the remedy.

The second potency (2 or 2c) is obtained by adding one drop of the 1st potency to ninety nine drops of diluent and shaking about thirty times. The third potency (3 or 3c) is obtained in the same manner by adding a drop of the previous potency (2 or 2c) to ninety nine drops of diluent and shaking about thirty times. This process of adding one drop of the previous potency to ninety nine drops of diluent is repeated up to the two hundredth (200 or 200c), one thousandth (1m), ten thousandth (10m) and so on.

The remedies are also prepared on the decimal scale which is one drop of the original substance to nine drops of diluent giving the 1× potency. All remedies prepared on this scale are indicated by an '×' following the name of the remedy. Potencies of the centesimal scale are suggested in the following pages.

Although it seems impossible, the process of potentisation releases the latent power or energy in the remedies and the higher the potency the greater the power which enters the human economy and helps the healing processes. Potencies above the 30th (200, 1m, etc) should be prescribed with great care, and only those with experience should use them.

The potencies and dosage suggested in this book are safe but they are intended only as a guide, both may be varied according to the preference of the prescriber but they should not be used above the 30th by those without a sound knowledge of the basic principles of homoeopathy.

# WHERE TO OBTAIN THE REMEDIES

It is advisable to procure remedies from a chemist specializing in homoeopathy to be certain that they have been properly potentised from the correct original substances and carefully stored. There are a number of homoeopathic chemists offering an excellent postal service:

Ainsworth's Homoeopathic Pharmacy,
38 New Cavendish Street, London, W1M 7LH
(telephone 071-935 5330)
which holds the royal appointment.

Galen Homoeopathics,
Lewell Mill, Dorchester, Dorset DT2 8AN
(telephone 0305 63996)

E. Gould & Son Ltd,
14 Crowndale Road, London, NW1 1TT
(telephone 071-388 4752)

A. Nelson & Co.,
73 Duke Street, London, W1M 6BY
Mail order: 5 Endeavour Way, Wimbledon,
London, SW19 9UH
(telephone 081-946 8527)

Other sources of homoeopathic remedies are:

Freeman's, 7 Eaglesham Road, Clarkston, Glasgow

Helios Homoeopathic Pharmacy, 92 Camden Road, Tunbridge Wells, Kent

P.A. Janssen, 28 Ampthill Road, Bedford

Weleda (UK) Ltd, Heanor Road, Ilkeston, Derbyshire

In the U.S.A. one should contact:

John A. Bornemann & Sons,
1208 Amosland Road, Norwood, PA 19074

Formur Inc.,
4200 Laclede Avenue, St Louis, MO 63108

Homoeopathic Educational Services,
2124 Kittredge Street, Berkeley, CA 94704

Boericke & Tafel,
1011 Arch Street, Philadelphia, PA 19107

Standard Homoeopathic Co,
P.O. Box 61067, Los Angeles, CA 90061

In Canada:

Thompson's Homoeopathic Supplies,
844 Yonge Street, Toronto, Ont. M4W 2H1

Some chemists can supply a case to hold ten or twelve remedies for those who wish to build up a stock in order to be able to deal with any emergency without loss of time.

The frequency of the dose must be controlled by the potency and the extent of the trouble. In an emergency the remedy may be repeated every few minutes but **always lengthen the time between doses as improvement takes place.**

Remember that the higher the potency the deeper its action and it should not be repeated as frequently as remedies of lower potencies (6 and 12).

Homoeopathic remedies are available in pill, tablet and liquid form. There is absolutely no difference in their action.

The dose is one pill, tablet or drop; more would not increase its effect.

It is important to allow the remedy to dissolve under the tongue, never take with food or liquid and especially avoid swallowing with a drink.

When a patient is unable to deal with the remedy in solid form, dissolve 2 pills or crushed tablets in half-a-tumbler of cold water and give a teaspoonful as a dose.

Homoeopathic remedies must be treated with care as they are susceptible to outside influences such as heat, strong sunlight, and perfumes such as scent, soaps, lipstick etc. Store in a cool, dark place, ideally in a drawer or cupboard away from these bad influences.

# SECTION 1

### Abscess

In the early stages where there is severe pain, redness and throbbing, BELLADONNA 6 every two hours, less frequently as improvement sets in. When pus has formed, HEPAR SULPH 6 every two hours until it either discharges or disappears.

After discharge SILICA 6 three times a day for up to 3 days.

Bathing with CALENDULA lotion (20 drops of the ∅ in a wine glass of hot water) three times a day helps to prepare the tissues for opening and subsequent healing.

Any abscess on a gland should be dealt with by a doctor.

### Accidents

The first remedy to think of after any kind of accident is ARNICA because not only does it relieve the bruising of the 'soft' parts, flesh or muscle, but it removes the shock caused by accidents and this is very important. Shock always follows an accident even if there is not much physical injury and when this is removed the patient recovers so much more quickly.

ARNICA 30 should be in every home. One pill should be given immediately after any accident and this can be repeated at 15 minute intervals in serious conditions until professional help arrives. For less serious conditions a dose half-hourly for 2 or 3 doses may be administered but the frequency of doses must be determined by the condition of the patient. As symptoms improve the time between doses must always be lengthened. Other remedies may be needed after ARNICA, such as HYPERICUM, LEDUM, RUTA etc., which come under the appropriate headings.

## Appendicitis

Any sudden severe pain in the abdomen should always be suspected as appendicitis and a doctor should be consulted because complications can have grave consequences.

Should the services of a physician be unavailable or much delayed (which is unlikely), IRIS TENAX is the most specific remedy for appendicitis and covers great pain in that area, great tenderness to pressure on one spot with a deathly sensation in the pit of the stomach. Anything between the 3× and 30th potencies may be given, one pill 2 hourly.

Never administer any purgative.


## Apprehension

Before a race, examination, driving test, speech etc., a dose of ARGENTUM NITRICUM 30 an hour before and another just before the event. If the 30th potency is not available the 12th to be taken one hour, half-an-hour and just before the event.

Where the apprehension is accompanied by fear and trembling GELSEMIUM 12 or 30 in the same dosage.

Lack of confidence combined with apprehension before an event can be overcome by ANACARDIUM 30 an hour before and another just before the ordeal. This remedy is helpful when the mind goes blank during an examination.

## Asthma

Chronic asthma is a deep-seated disease needing constitutional treatment by an experienced homoeopath but an ACUTE ATTACK can often be helped by one of the following remedies. A dose may be given every fifteen minutes until there is improvement and then less frequently.

ARNICA 6 or 12 when the attack is caused by exertion, speaking etc. breathing is laboured or oppressed with shooting pains in chest.

ARSENICUM ALBUM 6 or 12 where there is anxiety with restlessness; uneasy tossing about; worse when lying down and on movement. Burning heat in chest; cold sweats and prostration. Attack usually worse after midnight. This remedy is often of help to elderly sufferers.

IPECACUANHA 6 or 12 for a tight feeling around the chest, panting and rattling in windpipe which feels full of mucus. There is gasping for breath; face is pale and feet cold; a troublesome cough but patient is unable to bring up any mucus.

LOBELIA INFLATA 6 or 12 for nervous asthma with constrictive, suffocative feeling; nausea; giddiness; vomiting; spasmodic cough.

NUX VOMICA 6 or 12 where an attack is brought on by a stomach upset through indiscrete eating or drinking. Usually occurs in the early morning. Patient is very irritable.

SAMBUCUS 6 or 12 is especially useful for children. Attack begins in night; there is sweat on throat and neck.

## Black Eye

ARNICA 30 should be given at hourly intervals for 4 or 5 doses but if bruising is relieved by cold applications (and this is often the case) LEDUM 30 hourly for 3 or 4 doses.

If there is pain in the eye-ball SYMPHYTUM 30 at hourly intervals for 3 or 4 doses.

## Blisters

Apply CALENDULA ointment or, if this is not available, bathe with a solution of 10 drops of CALENDULA $\emptyset$ in a wineglass of water.

Internally CAUSTICUM 12 or 30 night and morning, reduce dosage as improvement sets in.

## Boils

BELLADONNA 6 every two hours at commencement of trouble, the boil is red, hot, painful.

GUNPOWDER 3× a tablet every three hours when there are no indications for the use of another remedy. It is an excellent blood clearer.

HEPAR SULPH. 6 or 12 every three hours to hasten suppuration.

SILICA 6 every three hours when the boil is slow to mature.

TARENTULA CUBENSIS 6 or 12 every four hours. Dr Dorothy Shepherd seldom used any other remedy, she found that it was almost a specific for boils. The indications are very acute pain, inflammation, severe stinging, burning and throbbing. Boils usually of a purplish colour.

Externally 10 drops of HYPERICUM $\emptyset$ in a wineglass of tepid water and bathe three or four times a day.

ARNICA 6 one dose for a week or two will often act as a preventative where there is a tendency to this trouble.

## Bruised Bones (see Accidents)

After ARNICA if bones are bruised RUTA 6 or 12 three times a day for a few days.

If an injury was sustained months or even years ago and the bone is still painful RUTA 30 night and morning for one week. This prescription may be repeated after a month if the trouble has not completely cleared.

## Burns

Serious burns should always be under the care of skilled medical attention. Do not delay in obtaining help for severe burns.

A dose of ARNICA 30 should always be given immediately to allay shock. If there is fright as well as shock ACONITE 30 in the place of ARNICA.

To relieve pain CANTHARIS 30, a dose whenever the pain returns. If this remedy is not available URTICA URENS 30 will act in a similar manner.

Where pain is accompanied by restlessness and there are blisters CAUSTICUM 30, a dose every half-an-hour until the pain subsides, repeat only if the pain returns.

Externally URTICA URENS ∅ or HYPERICUM ∅, ten drops in a wineglass of water should be applied to the burn by dropping a little on to the sterile gauze or dressing covering the burn; do not remove the covering but keep it damp by applying more of the solution as soon as it is dry.

URTICA URENS ∅ should, at all times, be kept in the kitchen and applied to minor burns from stoves, irons etc. It relieves pain and prevents blistering. At the same time URTICA URENS 30 or CANTHARIS 30 may be given internally if the burn is severe, either will help to relieve pain, the dose can be given at half-hourly intervals, if necessary.

A blister should never be punctured unless it is absolutely necessary to relieve pain.

## Carbuncles

ANTHRACINUM 30 night and morning for a few days. The eruption is bluish with a very angry appearance and there is often a black centre. There is also intolerable burning.

BELLADONNA 6 or 12 every two hours where the carbuncle is shiny red, the pain is throbbing and stabbing, there can be drowsiness and an inability to sleep.

HEPAR SULPH. 6 or 12 every three hours if given early will sometimes abort the trouble, in the later stages it will promote suppuration.

SILICA 6 every three hours will promote suppuration, there is intense burning pain and the eruption is bluish-red.

TARENTULA CUBENSIS 6 or 12 every four hours. As in the case of boils Dr Dorothy Shepherd states that this remedy is almost specific, she prescribed it as a routine measure with great success. The indications for its use are usually burning, stinging, throbbing pain. The carbuncle is of a purplish colour.

The external application of HYPERICUM ∅ as recommended under 'Boils' is also helpful.

## Colic

One of the following may be given every fifteen minutes for up to three doses, then lengthen the time between doses as improvement takes place. If there is no improvement within a reasonable time seek professional help.

CHAMOMILLA 6 or 12 for much flatulence, abdomen distended like a drum. Drawing, tearing pains in abdomen. Griping in region of navel. Flatulent colic after anger. There is intolerance of pain, worse at night and by warmth.

COLCHICUM 6 or 12 for pain worse by eating, great

distension after taking flatulent food. Relief from bending double.

COLOCYNTH 6 or 12 for violent cutting pains relieved by pressure or bending double. Griping pain in intestines as if bowel was being squeezed. Colic very violent in paroxysms forcing patient to bend forward.

DIOSCOREA 6 or 12 for griping, drawing, bursting or cutting pains. Flatulent spasms worse by pressure and by doubling up, better by stretching, standing erect and walking about.

NUX VOMICA 6 or 12 for cramp-like pains in stomach. Pressure in stomach as if from a stone. Flatulent colic from use of improper food. Frequent desire for stool without effect. Irritability. This remedy is often indicated for persons who overeat and overdrink.

PLUMBUM 12 for violent colic radiating to all parts of the body. Abdominal wall feels drawn to the spine by a string. Abdomen hard as a stone. Obstinate constipation, faeces lumpy, packed together like sheep's dung.

VERATRUM ALBUM 6 or 12 for pain in abdomen as if cut with a knife. Cutting pains with violent nausea and vomiting. Intestines feel as if tied in knots. Cold sweat on forehead or over whole body. Great weakness with feeble pulse.

## Concussion

Severe cases must always be dealt with by skilled medical attention.

ARNICA 30 at half-hourly intervals for up to 6 doses where the trouble is not severe.

## Cramp

One of the following medicines may be taken at ten minute intervals for 3 or 4 doses, if necessary.

ARNICA 6 or 12 where pain in calves is caused by fatigue.

CUPRUM 6 or 12 for pain in feet and legs. Contraction of muscles and tendons.

LEDUM 12. This is often the most effective remedy and the only one necessary. If there is no obvious cause start with this and if it fails to give complete relief try CUPRUM.

NUX VOMICA 6 or 12 when the trouble is at night, in the calves and soles of the feet. Patient must stretch feet. Often helpful when there is no known cause.

RHUS TOX 6 or 12 where the trouble is in the daytime, only whilst sitting.

## Crushed Fingers and Toes

These parts are rich in nerve endings and, therefore, very sensitive.

HYPERICUM 30 has an affinity with the nerves and will afford prompt relief in injuries wherever they are involved. A dose as soon as possible after the injury and it can be repeated at 10 to 15 minute intervals but less often as the pain recedes.

An intercurrent dose of ARNICA 30 may be given for shock.

## Dental Troubles

ARNICA 12 or 30, a dose just before and immediately after an extraction or filling controls both the pain and bleeding. It can be repeated if the pain returns.

Where there is severe pain caused by damage to nerves HYPERICUM 30 at half-hourly intervals for a few doses will give relief. Stop taking the remedy as soon as the pain has eased.

Excessive nervousness and fearfulness before a visit to the dentist ACONITE 30 should be taken one hour before and another a few minutes before the treatment.

Nervousness with shaking and diarrhoea GELSEMIUM 30 as prescribed for ACONITE.

If either ACONITE or GELSEMIUM is given ARNICA may still be taken as advised above.

Great sensitivity to pain, especially in children, CHAMOMILLA 12 or 30 just before treatment.

If allergic to the anaesthetic, the heartbeat is fast and there is weakness of the legs, CHAMOMILLA 30 before the visit and another 3 doses at hourly intervals afterwards helps to restore calm.

Sharp darting pains from drilling, HYPERICUM 30 for up to 3 doses at hourly intervals.

Excessive bleeding can be controlled by PHOSPHORUS 30, 3 doses at hourly intervals.

A mouth wash of 10 drops of CALENDULA Ø in half-a-tumbler of water will promote healing after an extraction but care should be taken to ensure that no chip of bone is left in the gum before its use as this powerful healing agent could heal over it and thus cause trouble. A mouthwash should not be used too frequently as there would be the risk of dislodging the blood clot.

**Diarrhoea**

One of the folllowing remedies may be taken at hourly intervals for 3 doses then less frequently as the condition improves. If the trouble does not clear up within a reasonable time seek expert advice.

ALOE 6 for constant urging to stool but there is uncertainty whether flatus or stool will be passed. After passing stool there is prostration accompanied by sweating.

ARSENICUM ALBUM 6 or 12 when caused by tainted foods, excessive amounts of fruit, especially melon, also ice cream or ice cold drinks when hot. Nausea, vomiting, restlessness, heat in stomach, burning sensation when expelling stool. Extreme weakness and coldness of extremities are pointers to this remedy.

CHINA 6 or 12 for frequent watery stools with much flatus, usually painless but sometimes there is a griping pain. Summer diarrhoea. Food is passed undigested. Diarrhoea after food. Often there is great debility.

COLOCYNTH 6 for watery, saffron yellow stools, after eating or drinking. Colic relieved by pressure and bending.

DULCAMARA 6 or 12 for sudden attacks caused by change of weather from hot to cold or from getting wet. Stools slimy green or yellow. Colic with feeling as though diarrhoea would occur. Loss of appetite and thirst.

PODOPHYLLUM 6 or 12 for profuse, watery, yellow offensive stools, gushing and painless. They often occur in the early morning or after eating. There may be cramps which are relieved by heat and bending double. Weak feeling in the abdomen.

VERATRUM ALBUM 6 or 12 for summer diarrhoea that is frequent, profuse and watery, with colic and cramps, great thirst for very cold water or acid drinks. Violent nausea with frothy vomiting. Sinking and empty feeling in stomach after stool. Icy cold sweat.

Diarrhoea from the use of antibiotics. NITRIC ACID 30 is almost a specific. A dose every 2 hours will often produce a rapid improvement. Stools slimy and offensive. Afterwards irritable and exhausted.

## Earache

Select the most appropriate remedy from the following and give a dose at hourly intervals for up to 3 doses, less frequently as improvement sets in. After the third dose the remedy may be given at 2 hourly intervals for another 3 doses and subsequently 3 times a day. If the trouble does not clear up or show great improvement within a reasonable time seek professional advice.

ACONITE 6 or 12 after exposure to cold or cold winds and where there is fever, restlessness and anxiety. Violent pain is sometimes relieved by heat.

BELLADONNA 6 or 12 for sudden onset of throbbing pain more frequently on the right side. Skin dry and face red and hot. Burning skin. There is restlessness. Patient is thirstless.

CHAMOMILLA 6 or 12 when the patient is very sensitive to pain which induces irritability. Pain worse from warm applications. Child very cross and fretful. Sometimes one cheek red and hot, the other pale and cold.

FERRUM PHOS. 6 or 12 is most helpful in the early stages of earache where there is inflammation.

HEPAR SULPH. 6 or 12 for stitching pains, patient is worse from draughts and wishes to be well wrapped up. Sensitive to touch.

MERCURIUS SOL. 30 is very helpful when there is inflammation of the middle ear. A dose 2 hourly but reducing to 4 hourly and then 3 times daily as symptoms improve.

PULSATILLA 6 or 12 for severe throbbing, ears feel as if they are stopped up. Worse from warmth, in the evening and at night. Patient is very weepy and wants sympathy. Craves fresh air.

Never put anything in the ear.

## Fainting

Place patient flat on back, head low, loosen tight clothing around neck and waist.

Select a remedy from the following and give at half-hourly intervals. If necessary more frequently.

From grief or emotional upset, IGNATIA 30.

From excitement, COFFEA 30.

From hot, stuffy atmosphere, PULSATILLA 30.

From pain, ACONITE 30 or CHAMOMILLA 30, whichever is at hand.

From sight of blood, NUX VOMICA 30.

From loss of blood, CHINA 30.

If the remedy is required in liquid form dissolve 2 pills or crushed tablets in half-a-glass of cold water. Even a few drops will suffice as a dose.

### Falls (see Accidents)

ARNICA 30 to allay shock. Repeat at half-hourly intervals for 3 doses, if necessary, but less often as symptoms improve.

If there is any physical damage see treatment under the appropriate heading.

### Food Poisoning

This can be quite serious and a doctor should be called but ARSENICUM ALB. 30 at hourly intervals for 3 or 4 doses will often clear up food or ptomaine poisoning if given after vomiting and diarrhoea have started. Patient is often restless and anxious.

If poison occurs from tainted fish then CARBO VEG. 30 given in the same dosage will alleviate the symptoms.

### Fractures (see Accidents)

Fractures must always be dealt with by a surgeon.

SYMPHYTUM 12 three times a day for 2 weeks or SYMPHYTUM 30 night and morning for the same period will reduce pain and speed up the knitting of bones.

CALC PHOS. 6× may be given for a further 4 weeks, if necessary.

### Grazes

Clean the wound gently with a solution of 10 drops of

CALENDULA ∅ in half-a-glass of water. Cover but keep the bandage moist by pouring a few drops of the liquid over it as soon as it begins to dry out. Healing should take place quickly.

## Grief

Grief affects many people at some time in their lives and if not dispelled it can lead to many physical symptoms.

IGNATIA is usually the first remedy to be thought of where there is either silent brooding or sadness and tears, even hysteria. A dose of the 30th potency 3 times daily for 1 week is usually very helpful.

NATRUM MURIATICUM 30 when very depressed from grief and consolation aggravates. Must be alone to cry. Dosage same as for IGNATIA.

ACID PHOS. 30 for debility from grief, listlessness, apathy, indifference, despairing. A dose 3 times daily for 1 week.

## Headache

One of the following medicines may be taken at 15 minute intervals for 3 or 4 doses, if necessary.

ACONITE 6 or 12 for sudden violent pain with burning sensation as if the brain were agitated by boiling water. Intolerable pain. Front of head as if nailed up. Feeling as if the whole head would be pushed through the forehead. Throbbing in temples going from one side to the other. Patient restless, thirsty and fearful.

ARSENICUM ALBUM 6 or 12 for periodic headache, often caused or accompanied by debility. Beating pain in forehead with inclination to vomit. Violent vomiting often after eating or drinking. Great thirst, drinks little but often. Restlessness. Prostration. Fear of death. Pains worse when at rest, better by motion.

BELLADONNA 6 or 12 for violent headache that comes on suddenly. Throbbing, bursting pain worse movement, stooping, moving the eyes. Hammering pains. Head hot, face flushed. Pain starts suddenly and ceases abruptly. Sometimes over the whole head or in the temples. Cannot bear noise or bright light. Worse from lying down. Often begins in afternoon and lasts all night.

These headaches can come on from exposure either to the sun or shock or emotions or periods. They often develop after washing the hair and not drying it properly or after a hair cut.

These can be chilly patients and in spite of intense heat in the head they like to be wrapped up.

GELSEMIUM 6 or 12 for a very bad headache that comes on with the flu or some acute disease or sometimes from great strain and anxiety.

Begins in the nape of the neck and settles over eyes which feel heavy and there is always haziness or some disturbance in vision before a headache. Boring pain over right eye especially or frontal. Comes on early or during the day and lasts until bedtime. Face is flushed, patient feels heavy, drowsy and sleepy. There are often shivers up and down the spine. Better after a good sleep. Vomiting as headache subsides. Patient passes much urine which alleviates. There is no thirst.

GLONOINE 6 or 12 for violent, pulsating, throbbing or bursting headache aggravated by light and bending head backwards. Nearly always caused by exposure to the sun or heat on head. Patient sits in chair holding head. Cannot bear any heat around head. Face flushed and head hot. Least jar or motion aggravates. Better cold air and cold applications. Sees different colours when looking at things.

NATRUM MURIATICUM 6 or 12 for beating in head as if from little hammers. Sharp stitches about head and sore, bruised feeling about eyeballs, worse when moved. Starts in back of neck and spreads all over the head. Blinding headache. Throbbing. Worse motion, warmth, using eyes and at the seaside. Often pre-menstrual, or after mental exertion or excitement.

NUX VOMICA 6 or 12 for stabbing pain with vomiting and nausea often caused by over indulgence in rich food or drink. Splitting headache as if a nail had been driven through the brain. Wakens feeling awful. Worse any conversation, mental excitement, movement (a picture of the 'morning after the night before'). Very irritable, very chilly. Nearly always constipated.

This remedy is often effective in those following a sedentary occupation.

PULSATILLA 6 or 12 for pain in temples and throbbing all over the head; head hot, relieved by cold applications. Periodic sick headache. Often associated with delayed, scanty or suppressed menses. Tearing, drawing or stitching pains worse towards evening. Vertigo when stooping or looking up. Often caused by rich, greasy foods. Patient is weepy, craves fresh air, better from walking slowly in air and from pressure. Worse stuffy atmosphere, lying down, stooping, in evening. Not thirsty.

SANGUINARIA 6 or 12 for sick headache beginning in morning and increasing in intensity during the day. Pains in back of head running in rays from neck upwards, settling over the right eye, with nausea, vomiting and dizziness. Patient lies still in a dark room. Worse from motion, stooping, noise and light.

## Heatstroke

Reduce the temperature by cold sponging in a cool, shady spot or room. Select one of the following remedies and give a dose at half-hourly intervals for up to 3 doses.

BELLADONNA 30 for dilated pupils, bounding pulse, burning, hot, dry skin with delirium.

BRYONIA 30 for splitting headache, worse on movement, with nausea, worse sitting up.

CUPRUM 30 for trouble accompanied by severe cramps.

GLONOINE 30 for throbbing, bursting headache, flushed face and sweaty skin.

## Insect Bites and Stings

Bathe the part affected with URTICA URENS ∅ or LEDUM ∅.

Internally LEDUM 30 at half-hourly intervals for up to 6 doses but lengthen the time between doses as improvement sets in. The indications for the use of this remedy are numbness, sensitivity to touch and pain better by cold applications.

Should LEDUM fail to relieve within a reasonable time give one of the following according to the symptoms, in the same dosage. This remedy has a very wide range of action in this field.

APIS 30 for burning, stinging pains aggravated by heat. The part swells rapidly and is rosy red (not bright red). There is puffiness rather than a hard swelling.

CANTHARIS 30 for very red inflammation with burning sensation that is worse from touch but relieved by gentle massage.

Both ARNICA ∅ and CALENDULA ∅ will give relief if the sting is bathed with the liquid.

Stings can occasionally cause very serious symptoms and a doctor should be consulted if the remedies do not control the trouble within a reasonable time.

## Nappy Rash

In fat children this may be caused by friction of two folds of skin, plastic or waterproof pants can be another cause. Always allow the baby to crawl about with a bare bottom several times a day to allow air to get to the parts and apply CALENDULA ointment.

Make sure the baby is well dried and if washable, always

rinse nappies in several lots of water after using a detergent.

## Nose Bleed

If caused by a blow or injury ARNICA 12 every few minutes until improvement, then less frequently.

For profuse nose bleeding (sometimes caused by vigorous blowing) PHOSPHORUS 12, a dose immediately and repeat every few minutes for 3 doses, if necessary.

VIPERA 12 in the same dosage is also very effective.

If the above mentioned remedies are not available try FERRUM PHOS. 12 in the same dosage.

## Sea Sickness

Poor sailors should take COCCULUS INDICUS 12 or 30 half-an-hour and again a few minutes before sailing as a preventative. If necessary, take at half-hourly intervals afterwards. The indications for the use of this remedy are great nausea, vertigo, faintness and loss of orientation.

PETROLEUM 12 is another most effective remedy for persistent nausea and an accumulation of water in the mouth, vomiting and giddiness better for eating. Worse from smell of petrol fumes.

TABACUM 12 is excellent for nausea, giddiness, vomiting, icy coldness, sinking feeling, worse for the smell of tobacco smoke.

The dosage for all remedies is the same as for COCCULUS INDICUS.

## Spine, Blow or Injury to Coccyx (base of spine) (see Accidents)

This is a particularly sensitive area with many nerve endings.

HYPERICUM 30 immediately, repeat night and morning

until pain subsides.

Where there is much bruising follow with ARNICA 30 night and morning but allow more time between doses as bruise improves.

If the bone is bruised RUTA 30 in the same dosage as ARNICA.

### Splinters

To expel deeply embedded splinters SILICA 6 three times a day, if unsuccessful within a few days obtain professional assistance.

UNDER NAIL. Seek professional help for removal and then apply CALENDULA Ointment. If this is not available use CALENDULA ∅, 10 drops in half-a-tumbler of water. Also take LEDUM 12 or 30 for 3 doses at four hourly intervals.

### Sprains

ARNICA 30 at hourly intervals for 4 or 5 doses should be given as soon as possible. If there is much improvement it may be continued at longer intervals between doses.

In bad sprains and where ARNICA does not clear up the trouble RHUS TOX. 6 or 12 three times daily should be given.

If the bone is painful RUTA 6 or 12, three times daily may be needed instead of RHUS TOX.

### Teething

Dissolve 2 pills or 2 crushed tablets in a quarter of a tumbler of warm water and administer a small teaspoonful as a dose.

One of the following may be given at quarter-of-an-hour intervals until the baby is peaceful.

BELLADONNA 6 or 12 when baby awakens in a fright with staring eyes. Starts and jumps during sleep. Face and eyes red, pupils dilated. Head hot. Restlessness. Feverishness. Convulsions followed by sound sleep. Gums swollen and inflamed.

CALC CARB. 6 or12 when there are head sweats during sleep. Peevishness. Fretfulness. Baby is a very light sleeper. Feet are cold and damp. Stools white or chalk like or thin and whitish. Vomiting of milk in thick curds. Swollen, distended abdomen.

CHAMOMILLA 6 or 12 is the most commonly used remedy for this complaint. Baby is very irritable, cross, peevish, never satisfied, when given something it is thrown to the floor. Wants to be carried all the time. Cries suddenly and tosses about during sleep. One cheek may be red, the other pale.

This remedy has saved numerous parents a sleepless night.

KREOSOTUM 6 or 12 is suitable for weak, delicate babies. There is painful, difficult dentition. Teeth decay as soon as they appear.

## Toothache

KREOSOTUM 3 given hourly cures many cases of toothache when there are no signs of inflammation or gumboils.

PLANTAGO 3 every 10 minutes if indications are not clear.

PLANTAGO ∅ may be rubbed on the gum around the painful tooth.

Where there is inflammation at the root of a decayed tooth, gums spongy, receding or they bleed easily, worse at night. Thirsty despite excessive salivation, MERC SOL. 6 at hourly intervals.

Where there is much swelling and inflammation in addition to pain, APIS 6 hourly.

Neuralgic pain, intolerable at night relieved by heat,

toothache in children while teething, MAG PHOS. 6 hourly.

Toothache better by holding cold water in the mouth, COFFEA 6 or 12 hourly.

## Vomiting

One of the following may be given at hourly intervals for 3 doses, if necessary. If the condition fails to improve seek professional assistance.

ANTIMONIUM TART. 6 or 12 for nausea and vomiting with faintness and hot sweat on face. Disgust of food, frequent nausea but relief from vomiting. Vomiting of liquids as soon as taken followed by langour and drowsiness. Patient is thirstless.

BRYONIA 6 or 12 where there is vomiting of solid food but not of drink; first of bile then food. Must keep still, the least motion aggravates the nausea or provokes vomiting.

IPECACUANHA 6 or 12 for vomiting with constant nausea. Vomiting of large quantities of food, mucus, bile or sour fluid. Stomach feels relaxed as if hanging down. Tongue clean or only lightly coated.

NUX VOMICA 6 or 12 for nausea and vomiting after overloading the stomach with food or drink. Urge to vomit but cannot do so. Vomiting of sour smelling and sour tasting mucus. Stomach sensitive to pressure. Patient usually cold and irritable.

PULSATILLA 6 or 12 for vomiting from a chill in the stomach or from suppressed menses. Vomiting caused by a disordered stomach, too much pastry or fat foods. Vomiting of mucus, bile or bitter-sour fluid, often worse during evening or night. Sticky feeling in mouth, frequent desire to cleanse mouth with cold water.

## Whitlow

One of the following medicines may be given 3 times a day for three to four days but lengthen the time between doses as improvement sets in.

ARSENICUM ALBUM 6 or 12 for burning pain like fire. Whitlow is angry looking or black. Patient is anxious and restless, worse about midnight.

HEPAR SULPH. 6 or 12 for violent throbbing, heat and swelling. Whitlow is very sensitive to touch. This remedy is suitable for those with unhealthy skin which suppurates from every little injury. Suppuration is accelerated by this remedy.

MERCURIUS SOL. 12 at the beginning of the trouble will often prevent suppuration.

SILICA 6 or 12 for a deep-seated whitlow with excessive pain and swelling. Give when suppuration is imminent or where discharge is fetid, thin and watery.

After MERCURIUS it is often helpful to give a weekly dose of SULPHUR and SILICA in alternation to remove the tendency to this trouble. Each remedy in the 12th potency, once a week for about 4 doses each.

## Wounds

Cleanse and then soak a pad in a solution of 10 drops of CALENDULA Ø in half-a-glass of cold water and apply to the wound.

If the part can be kept bandaged do not remove but keep it damp by pouring a few drops of the solution over the bandage as soon as it starts to get dry.

Internally CALENDULA 30 three times a day will hasten healing.

Extensive wounds should receive expert attention as they might need stitching, consult a doctor if in doubt, but CALENDULA 30 as recommended above will help even the most severe damage.

# SECTION 2

## SOME MOST IMPORTANT
## SYMPTOMS OF THE REMEDIES

### ACID PHOS.
Weakness of both mind and body often leading to nervous exhaustion.
Effects of acute disease, physical excesses, grief, mental shock.
Drowsy, apathetic.
Too fast growth, too tall growth.
Worse: bad news; draughts; winds.
Better: after short sleep.

### ACONITE
Fear is a leading characteristic – fear of death; crowds; anything.
Always anxious.
Physical and mental restlessness.
Acute and sudden onset of symptoms often caused by exposure to cold dry weather.
Worse: in warm room; in evening and early part of night; lying on affected side; from dry cold winds.
Better: in open air.

### ALOE
Abdomen feels full, heavy, hot and bloated.

37

Rectum feels weak with a sense of insecurity.
Burning in anus and rectum.
Worse: in early morning; heat; in hot, dry weather; after eating or drinking.
Better: from cold, open air.

## ANACARDIUM

Impaired memory, loss of memory, brain-fag, lack of self-confidence.
Of help in neurasthenia.
Pain in stomach only when empty, relieved by eating.
Worse: on application of hot water.
Better: from eating.

## ANTHRACINUM

Septic inflammations, boils and carbuncles.

## ANTIMONIUM TARTARICUM

Rattling of mucus but little expectoration.
Great drowsiness.
Debility.
Cold sweat.
Worse: in evening; lying down at night; from warmth.
Better: from sitting erect; from eructation and expectoration.

## APIS

Awkward, drops things readily.
Burning, stinging pains.
Much oedema.
Worse: heat in any form; touch; pressure; after sleep.
Better: in open air; uncovering, cold bathing.

## ARGENTUM NITRICUM

Fearful, anxious, nervous, impulsive.
A great remedy for anticipation, time passes too slowly,

must walk fast.
Examination funk.
Loathes heights, can be claustrophobic.
Great desire for sweets.
Cannot stand heat.
Worse: warmth in any form; at night; sweats; after eating.
Better: fresh air; cold; from eructations.

## ARNICA

The first remedy to be thought of in accidents, takes away the shock which is always present in accidents.
Bruises of the flesh.
Relieves sore, bruised feeling caused by injury. Bed feels hard.
Weakness, weariness, sensation as of being bruised.
Wants to be left alone, always says he is all right no matter how ill.

## ARSENICUM ALBUM

Restlessness, burning, prostration, after midnight.
Great anxiety, fear, restlessness often driving the patient from place to place.
Great exhaustion after even slight exertion.
Very chilly.
Fastidious and exacting.
Thirsty, but drinks little at a time.
Worse: from cold air; cold applications; at night; after midnight.
Better: warmth; hot applications. Although patient is better by warmth a headache is better by cold.

## BELLADONNA

Acute inflammatory troubles with pain, redness of skin, puffiness. Eyes staring, bloodshot with dilated pupils.
Great sensitivity to pain and motion. Pains appear suddenly and disappear just as suddenly.

Skin very red and hot, radiates heat.
Worse: after 3 p.m. or after midnight, from uncovering, or or draught of air; lying down.
Better: from covering; holding head high.

## BRYONIA

A most valuable pointer to the use of this remedy is that all troubles are aggravated by motion.
Patient is easily irritated or angered and is often spare and dark complexioned.
Great dryness of all mucous membranes.
Anxiety about the future, a great sense of insecurity.
Thirst for long drinks.
Worse: warmth; motion; hot weather; exertion; touch; in morning. Cannot sit up, gets faint and sick.
Better: lying on painful side; pressure; rest; cold things.

## CALCAREA CARBONICA

Often called for in patients who are fat, flabby, inclined to obesity.
There is coldness, often a feeling of wearing cold, damp socks or stockings.
Profuse sweats on head of children with fontanelles open, skull often very large.
Skin white or chalky pale.
Patient sluggish or slow in his movements.
Worse: from exertion, whether mental or physical; ascending; cold in every form; standing.
Better: dry climate and weather.

## CALCAREA PHOSPHORICA

Excellent for broken bones where they are slow to knit.
Tardy dentition.
Anaemic children who are peevish, have cold extremities and feeble digestion.
Worse: exposure to damp, cold weather.

Better: warm, dry atmosphere; in summer.

## CALENDULA
A wonderful remedy for cuts, incised wounds etc. When the $\emptyset$ is applied to such injuries it will stop the bleeding very quickly and promote healing.

## CANTHARIS
Burning is one of the great indications for this remedy; burning, cutting pains with frequent urge to urinate.
Excessive burning pain in eyes, mouth, throat, stomach etc., often accompanied by the urinary trouble mentioned above.
Burns, applied locally and internally.

## CARBO VEGETABILIS
Great accumulation of flatulence in stomach; stomach feels full and tense from flatulence.
People who have never recovered from the effects of a previous illness, there may be anaemia and depletion.
Acidity.
Temporary relief from belching.
Worse: evening; night; open air; cold; fat food; warm, damp weather; wine.
Better: from eructations; from fanning (when they need air); cold.

## CAUSTICUM
Burning, rawness and soreness of various parts, throat, larynx, chest, rectum etc.
Great weakness, sinking of strength, with trembling.
Drooping of eyelids.
Involuntary passage of urine when coughing, sneezing, blowing the nose, when walking, at night during sleep.
Worse: dry, cold winds; in fine weather; cold air.
Better: damp, wet weather; warmth; heat of bed.

41

## CHAMOMILLA

Great sensitivity to pain.

Irritability and crossness, child wants an object and then throws it away.

Ailments brought on by anger.

Restlessness and sleeplessness.

Pains with numbness.

Worse: by heat; anger; open air; wind; at night.

Better: from being carried; warm wet weather.

Mental calmness contra-indicates Chamomilla.

## CHINA

Debility and weakness after excessive loss of fluids, profuse suppuration, prolonged diarrhoea.

Dr H.N. Guernsey said 'Uncomfortable distention of the abdomen, with a wish to belch up, or a sensation as if the abdomen were packed full, not in the least relieved by eructation'.

Great sensitiveness, the slightest pressure will increase pain in an affected part, yet hard pressure will relieve.

Worse: slightest touch; draught of air; loss of vital fluids; after eating.

Better: bending double; hard pressure; open air; warmth.

## COCCULUS INDICUS

One of the great sickness remedies – sickness from riding in a car or boat.

Sensation of weakness or hollowness in various organs.

Ill effects from loss of sleep or over work.

Weakness of neck muscles with heaviness of head, muscles seem unable to support the head.

Vertigo on rising from bed compelling sufferer to lie down again.

In seasickness patient is better in fresh air.

Worse: eating; after loss of sleep; open air; smoking; riding; noise.

## COFFEA

All senses are more acute – smell, taste and touch.

Great activity of mind, head full of ideas; active brain causes sleeplessness.

Troubles from sudden surprises, patient is very emotional.

Very sensitive to pain.

An unusual symptom is a jerking toothache relieved by ice cold water.

Worse: excessive emotions (joy); strong odours; noise; open air; cold; night.

Better: warmth; from lying down; holding ice in mouth.

## COLCHICUM

The smell of food cooking nauseates to faintness.

Bloating and distension of the abdomen.

Dyspepsia when there is burning or a sensation of coldness in stomach, often with much gas in stomach or abdomen.

Worse: from sundown to sunrise; motion; loss of sleep; smell of food in evening; mental exertion.

Better: stooping.

## COLOCYNTH

Severe colic relieved by bending double or pressing the abdomen against something hard. The pain is neuralgic in character, often accompanied by vomiting and diarrhoea.

Cramp-like pain in sciatic nerve better from pressure and heat, worse when still.

Worse: from anger; after eating.

Better: from doubling up; hard pressure; warmth; lying with head bent forward.

## CUPRUM

Spasms often beginning by twitching in the fingers and toes and spreading from there.

Cramps or convulsions.

Worse: from vomiting; contact.

Better: during perspiration; drinking cold water.

## DIOSCOREA

Colic pain in navel area radiating to all parts, worse from bending, better standing erect.
Rumbling in the bowels, passing of much flatus.
Worse: lying down; doubling up; in evening and night.
Better: standing erect; motion in open air; pressure.

## DULCAMARA

Complaints caused or aggravated by change of weather from warm to cold.
Stiff neck, painful back, limbs lame, sore throat and quinsy.
Stiff tongue and jaws.
Worse: from cold in general; damp, rainy weather; at night; at rest.
Better: motion; dry weather; external warmth.

## FERRUM PHOSPHORICUM

Early stages of a cold without definite symptoms calling for another remedy.
Haemorrhages including nose bleed – blood is bright red.
Frontal headache followed and relieved by nose bleed.
Fever, skin hot and dry.
Worse: at night; between 4 to 6 a.m.; touch; jar; motion; right side.
Better: cold applications.

## GELSEMIUM

Excellent 'flu remedy where there is complete relaxation of the muscles, weakness and trembling of limbs, chills run up and down the spine. Even the eyelids droop.
Dull, tired headache.
Mental faculties dull, patient unable to think clearly or fix his attention.
Susceptibility to mental disturbance such as sudden

excitement, emotion, fright etc.

Worse: damp weather; fog; before a thunderstorm; emotion; excitement; bad news.

Better: bending forward; profuse urination; open air; continued motion.

## GLONOINE

Bursting headache rising from the neck with great throbbing; patient carries the head carefully as he cannot bear the least jar.

Cannot bear anything on head.

Sunstroke and troubles caused by overheating.

Worse: in sun; exposure to sun-rays, gas, open fire; jar; stooping; having hair cut; stimulants; lying down; from 6 a.m. to noon; left side.

Better: brandy.

## GUNPOWDER

An excellent blood clearer.

Boils and carbuncles.

## HEPAR SULPHURIS

Great sensitivity to touch, pain, cold air; patient can faint with pain.

Even slight scratches or injuries suppurate.

Unhealthy skin, very slow to heal.

Sour diarrhoea; a child often smells sour.

Boils, abscesses. Hastens suppuration when pus has formed.

Worse: from exposure to dry, cold air and winds; cool air; slightest draught; touch; lying on painful side.

Better: in damp weather; from wrapping up head; warmth; after eating.

## HYPERICUM

Injuries to nerves; toes, fingers and the base of the spine

(Coccyx).
Puncture wounds from nails, splinters, pins, stings and bites.
The Ø diluted in water can be applied externally to supplement internal medication.

## IGNATIA

Ailments caused by grief, shock, fright, disappointment.
Has helped a vast number of people in a despondent condition caused by the loss of a wife, husband or loved one.
Much sighing, sobbing, sadness from suppressed grief.
Changeable, moody disposition.
Headaches when there is a sensation as if a nail were driven through the side of the head, relieved by lying on it.
Extreme aversion to tobacco smoke.
Worse: in the morning; open air; after meals; coffee; smoking; liquids; external warmth.
Better: while eating; change of position.

## IPECACUANHA

The chief feature is persistent nausea and vomiting, the patient is thirstless.
Stomach and bowels feel as if they are hanging down.
Diarrhoea, stools green and slimy, coming in gushes with great straining and prostration.
Hacking cough caused by a tickle in trachea which causes a feeling of nausea and suffocation often accompanied by vomiting.
Cough incessant and violent, chest seems full of mucus.
Worse: periodically; moist warm wind; lying down.

## IRIS TENAX

A remedy for appendicitis.
Headache in temples with vomiting of green bile.

## KREOSOTUM

Tendency to haemorrhage; small wounds bleed profusely.
Excoriating, burning and offensive discharges.
Gums painful, dark red or blue. Teeth decay as soon as they appear.
Copious pale urine. Great and sudden urge to urinate.
Child wets bed during first sleep.
Worse: in open air; cold; rest; when lying; after menstruation.
Better: from warmth; motion; warm diet.

## LEDUM

Puncture wounds from nails, pins, needles etc., especially when there is little bleeding. Part often becomes pale, cold and puffy.
Bites of animals – dogs, rats etc.
If shooting pains develop and lockjaw is threatened use Hypericum.
Tetanus with twitching of muscles near wound.
Black eye.
Rheumatism beginning in feet and travelling upwards, the swellings are pale.
Lack of body warmth, yet heat of bed intolerable.
Worse: at night; from heat of bed.
Better: from cold; uncovering; cold water – putting feet in cold water gives relief.

## LOBELIA

Nausea and vomiting with relaxation of the muscular system and a profuse accumulation of saliva.
Bronchitis and asthma, chest oppressed as if full of blood which seems to stagnate.
Worse: motion; cold, especially cold washing; in afternoon; tobacco.
Better: from warmth; towards evening.

## MAGNESIA PHOSPHORICA

Cramping pains in any part of the body, sometimes caused by over-exertion.

Neuralgic and spasmodic pains, can be shooting, lightning-like or boring.

Infants cutting teeth, sometimes have spasms or convulsions without fever.

Worse: right side; cold; cold air; cold water; touch; at night.

Better: warmth; pressure; bending double; friction.

## MERCURIUS SOL.

Profuse, fetid sweats which give no relief.

Offensive breath, spongy bleeding gums, flabby tongue with profuse salivation.

Trembling of limbs.

Creeping chilliness at onset of disease.

Worse: at night; wet, damp weather; lying on right side; perspiring; warm room; warm bed.

## NATRUM MURIATICUM

Patients are melancholy and irritable but consolation or fuss aggravates. There is usually an aggravation at the seaside but in a few cases there is amelioration.

Great desire for salt and dislike of fat.

Wind and laughter make the eyes water.

Cannot urinate in the presence of other people.

Hang nails. Skin around nails dry and cracked.

Numbness and tingling in fingers and toes.

Great emaciation in spite of good appetite, showing most around the neck.

Great dryness of mucous membranes, lips dry and cracked, especially in middle.

Worse: noise; music; in warm room; lying down; about 10 a.m.; at seaside; mental exertion; consolation; heat; talking.

Better: in open air; cold bathing; going without regular meals; lying on right side; tight clothing.

## NITRIC ACID

Cracks, warts, ulcers and fissures surrounding any orifice.
Sticking pain as if from a splinter in any affected part.
Craving for fat and salt and substances containing lime.
Aversion to meat and bread.
Urine strong smelling, like horses urine.
Warts sensitive and bleed easily.
Profuse cold sweat of hands and feet.
Patient is chilly, nervous, irritable, indifferent.
Worse: in evening and at night; cold climate, also in hot weather; noise; jar.
Better: whilst travelling in any vehicle.


## NUX VOMICA

Often needed in the treatment of people (more often men) who lead sedentary lives, sitting at a desk all day, and those who habitually over-eat and over-drink. They are irritable, spiteful, malicious, inclined to get angry or are easily offended.

Their over-indulgence in excessive rich or highly seasoned food causes them to wake about 3 a.m., and then they find it difficult to get off to sleep again. When they eventually fall asleep they are reluctant to get up, are tired, irritable, with sour breath and feel poorly.

In constipation there is a frequent but ineffective desire to pass stool, or very small quantities are passed at each attempt.

Patients are very chilly and when ill are unable to get warm even though they hug a fire. In bed the slightest movement of the clothes makes them feel cold.

Vomiting from a sour stomach with much retching and straining. Bitter, putrid taste in mouth.

An excellent remedy for 'The morning after the night before'.

Worse: morning; mental exertion; after eating; touch; spices; stimulants; dry weather; cold.

Better: from a nap if allowed to complete it; in evening while at rest; damp, wet weather; strong pressure.

## PETROLEUM

One of the leading seasickness remedies.

Eczema on various parts of the body. Chaps on hands which bleed. All are worse in the winter and better or disappear in the summer.

Colic followed by diarrhoea, but only in the daytime.

Chilblains which are moist, burn and itch in cold weather.

Even slight scratches or abrasions suppurate.

Worse: dampness; before and during thunderstorm; from riding in cars, passive motion; in winter; from mental states.

Better: warm air; dry weather; lying with head high.

## PHOSPHORUS

Patients needing this remedy are usually tall, slender, narrow chested with fine skin, soft hair, long silky lashes. Complexion changeable with easy flushing of the face.

Mentally they are sensitive with an active imagination, fearful of thunderstorms, of being alone, of the dark, worse at twilight until midnight.

Burning pains in various parts; heat running up the back.

Patients crave cold drinks, food, ice cream etc., but as soon as the liquid becomes warm in the stomach it is vomited.

Hunger, people often get up in the night to eat. Are often hungry soon after eating a meal.

Haemorrhage, small bleeding of bright blood from nose, anus.

Diarrhoea, stool watery and profuse, pouring away as though anus were constantly wide open.

Worse: touch; physical and mental exertion; twilight; evening; warm food and drink; change of weather; from getting wet in hot weather; lying on left or painful side; during a thunderstorm; ascending stairs.

Better: in dark; lying on right side; cold; cold food; open air; washing in cold water; sleep.

## PLANTAGO

Helpful in toothache, a low potency (say 3rd) internally and the ∅ rubbed around the painful tooth.

## PLUMBUM

Violent colic accompanied by extreme constipation. There is a feeling as if the abdomen were pulled towards the spine by a string.

Patients are often very slow in their movements and reactions, have pallied yellowish complexions, shrivelled, dry, wrinkled skin. Are emaciated with sunken cheeks and often anaemic.

Depressed, sad people with bad memories. Emotional and, at times, hysterical.

There is a blue line along the margin of the gums.

Worse: at night; motion.

Better: rubbing; hard pressure; physical exertion.

## PODOPHYLLUM

Diarrhoea which is offensive and seems to drain the patient dry and is often painless.

The diarrhoea often alternates with constipation, no stool being passed for days and then diarrhoea. Infants often roll their heads from side to side during sleep and make a chewing motion with their jaws. There is a desire to press the gums or teeth together.

The mental state is one of depression and melancholia; there is restlessness.

Worse: in early morning; in hot weather; during dentition.

## PULSATILLA

Patients requiring this remedy are often timid, gentle, of a yielding disposition, inclined to be fleshy. But others, although timid, gentle etc., are irritable, easily irritated, extremely touchy, always feel they are being slighted.

There is sadness and despondency, weeps easily.

The patient is chilly yet cannot bear heat in any form. Cannot stay in a warm stuffy room, must have plenty of fresh air, they feel better by moving about slowly.

There is dislike of sitting in the sun and patients feel worse for changes in the weather, in wet weather and by getting wet, especially the feet. There is also dislike of wind.

Aches and pains often move from place to place and a peculiarity is that symptoms often occur on one half of the body only; perspiration might be on one side of the face or body only.

Catarrhal discharge is thick greeny/yellow and bland.

Thirstlessness even in a fever. Cannot digest greasy and rich foods, cakes and pastry. There is dislike of hot food, a preference for everything cold and a desire for sour and refreshing foods.

Worse: from heat; rich fat food; after eating; towards evening; in a warm room; lying on left or painless side; when allowing feet to hang down.

Better: open air; motion; cold applications; cold food and drinks, though not thirsty.

## RHUS TOXICODENDRON

A remedy for sprains, acts on the fibrous and muscular tissues.

Rheumatism, lumbago, stiff neck, the pains are aggravated by cold and damp conditions.

Sitting or lying in one position causes stiffness and aching, the patient is compelled to move about or change position for relief; there is restlessness in bed, constant movement to ease the pain.

Worse: during sleep; cold, wet, rainy weather; after rain; cold bathing; sea bathing; at night; during rest; when lying on back or right side.

Better: warm, dry weather; motion; walking; change of position; rubbing; warm applications; from stretching out limbs.

## RUTA

Bruises of the bone, even very old injuries where there is still trouble in the bone will benefit from this remedy. There is a bruised, lame sensation.

Where there is pain in the wrists, worse in cold, wet weather and better by motion.

Eye-strain from close work, eyes feel weary and ache as if strained or burn like balls of fire.

Worse: lying down; from cold, wet weather.

## SAMBUCUS NIGRA

Snuffles in small children, the condition is dry yet the nose is completely obstructed. Child must breathe through the mouth.

In asthma attacks which come on suddenly in the night, the child turns blue and gasps for breath. After the attack the child goes to sleep and wakens with another attack and this is repeated.

Worse: sleep; during rest; after eating fruit.

Better: sitting up in bed; motion.

## SANGUINARIA

Sick headache commencing at back of head and spreading over head and settling over the right eye with nausea and vomiting. Patient wants to be in a dark room and perfectly quiet.

Loose cough with badly smelling sputa, breath even smells bad to the patient.

Rheumatic pain in the right arm and shoulder, worse at night.

Worse: sweets; right side; motion; touch.

Better: acids; sleep; darkness.

## SILICA

Chilly, undernourished patients (not from lack of nourishing food but assimilation), who are weak, nervous, faint-hearted, yielding, shy, timid, afraid to tackle anything for fear of failure.

Big head and tummy, body thin with soft bones, bad teeth and nails.

Offensive odour from feet, can be caused by suppressed sweat.

Boils, whitlows and septic conditions.

Has the power to push out foreign bodies such as splinters.

Wounds that fester, skin heals badly.

Worse: in morning; from washing; during menses; uncovering; lying down; lying on left side; cold; damp.

Better: warmth; wrapping up head; in summer; in wet or humid weather.


## SULPHUR

Burning is one of the important pointers to the use of this remedy; burning everywhere, in eyes, in face without redness, in tongue, in stomach etc.

All orifices are extremely red, lips, ears, tip of nose, anus, red rimmed eyes.

Burning hands and feet, has to put them out of bed to cool.

All complaints are worse from heat but they are, to a lesser degree, worse from cold, a moderate temperature is most suitable.

Skin troubles are common, there is excessive dryness and irritation. The intense itching compels scratching which does not relieve but is followed by burning. The skin looks dirty and washing does not help; it is rough and harsh.

Hair looks dry and forehead may be covered with blackheads or pimples.

Lazy, indolent people who find it difficult to stand for any length of time, they sink into a chair.

Empty, sinking feeling at mid-morning and if they do not

have something to eat there is weakness, faintness and even nausea.

Offensive body odour even nauseating the sufferer; washing does not have any effect.

Patient is usually slovenly, untidy and dislikes washing or bathing.

Worse: at rest; when standing; warmth of bed; washing; bathing; in morning at 11 o'clock; at night; from alcohol.

Better: dry warm weather; lying on right side; drawing up affected limbs.


## SYMPHYTUM

Speeds up knitting of bones.


## TABACUM

Seasickness where there is deathly nausea, pallor, coldness, better in cold fresh air.

Vertigo, death like pallor leading to loss of consciousness, better in open air and vomiting. Vertigo on opening the eyes.

Worse: opening eyes; in evening; extremes of heat and cold.

Better: uncovering; open fresh air.


## TARENTULA CUBENSIS

A most efficacious remedy for boils, abscesses, felons or swellings of any kind where the tissues are of a bluish colour and there are intense burning pains.

Worse: at night.

Better: smoking.


## URTICA URENS

An excellent remedy for burns.

Antidotes the effects of eating shell fish.

Worse: from snow-air; water; cool moist air; touch.

## VERATRUM ALBUM

Collapse or great coldness with cold sweat, especially on the forehead.

Violent purging and vomiting with profuse sweat.

Stools like rice water, profuse and exhausting.

Cramps in extremities.

Whole body icy cold. A craving for ice and ice cold water in spite of the coldness.

Worse: at night; wet, cold weather.

Better: walking; warmth.

## VIPERA

Nose bleed and haemorrhage.

Some readers may wish to delve more deeply into homoeopathy and there are many books on the subject. The following are recommended.

**HOMOEOPATHY AND IMMUNIZATION** by Leslie J. Speight. This small work gives details for the use of the homoeopathic prophylactics in epidemic diseases. The subject is of great topical interest and this is a book that should be studied by those wishing to avoid the dangers of crude immunizations.

**HOMOEOPATHY – A PRACTICAL GUIDE TO NATURAL MEDICINE** by Phyllis Speight. The most popular book for beginners covers much ground by explaining, in simple language, the basic principles and the treatment of many common ailments. This is highly recommended.

**PUDDEPHATT'S PRIMERS.** The author originally issued 3 booklets entitled 'First Steps to Homoeopathy', 'How To Find The Correct Remedy' and 'The Homoeopathic Materia Medica, How It Should Be Studied'. These booklets have been edited and condensed into one small book.

**HOMOEOPATHY FOR THE FIRST AIDER** by Dr Dorothy Shepherd. A most popular work giving advice for the use of the common remedies in various injuries and ailments. The author presents the facts in an interesting manner and gives details of some cases she treated successfully.

**HOMOEOPATHY IN EPIDEMIC DISEASES** by Dr Dorothy Shepherd. The author, a very widely experienced practitioner, emphasises the speed with which infectious diseases can be dealt with by the use of homoeopathic remedies. Not only can the troubles be overcome speedily, the suffering is reduced and there is no risk of side effects from the medicines.

**A STUDY COURSE IN HOMOEOPATHY** by Phyllis Speight. Originally issued as a correspondence course in 12 lessons which have been edited and now offered in book form. An excellent means of study for those seeking to learn the basic principles of homoeopathy.

Homoeopathy is also successful in dealing with animals and two books, **CATS: HOMOEOPATHIC REMEDIES** and **DOGS: HOMOEOPATHIC REMEDIES** by G. Macleod are intended for domestic use. Many people have expressed appreciation of the help derived from these books.

All the above are published by:

**Health Science Press**
**The C.W. Daniel Company Ltd**
**1 Church Path, Saffron Walden, Essex, England**

# INDEX